NAVIGATING GALLBLADDER CANCER WITH CONFIDENCE AND CARE

Mastering The Journey And Empowering Strategies For Quick Approach To Cancer Recovery For Relief And Vibrant Healing

DR. WESLEY IAN

DISCLAIMER

The information in this book is not meant to replace professional medical advice, diagnosis, or treatment; rather, it is meant mainly for general informational reasons. If you have any questions about a medical problem, you should always consult your doctor or another trained health expert. Don't ever discount expert medical advice or put off getting it because of something you've read in this book.

Any negative effects or repercussions arising from the usage of the material provided herein are not the responsibility of the book's author or publisher. It should be noted by readers that the material in this book is not all-inclusive and might not address every facet of the subject. Furthermore, new research may have an impact on how health concerns are understood or treated because medical knowledge is always changing.

No particular test, treatment, method, or product mentioned in this book is endorsed or promoted by the author or publisher. The reader assumes all risk associated with using the information included in this book.

Before making any big decisions regarding your health, it's crucial to speak with a licensed healthcare provider. The relationship between a patient and their healthcare practitioner should not be replaced by this book, nor is it meant to offer medical advice.

The opinions presented in this book are the author's and may not necessarily represent those of the publisher. Any errors, omissions, or inaccuracies in the information in this book are not the responsibility of the author or publisher.

It is recommended that readers independently confirm any information contained in this book and speak with a healthcare provider about their specific medical needs and state of health.

TABLE OF CONTENTS

ABOUT THE BOOK

"Navigating Gallbladder Cancer with Confidence and Care" is a priceless tool for people and families who are attempting to navigate the intricacies of gallbladder cancer. The book is significant because it takes a complete approach to empowering patients, caregivers, and healthcare professionals in equal measure. It is written with compassion and skill. Drawing from a wealth of experience, the author deftly tackles the complex issues of gallbladder cancer, offering a path forward that promotes comprehension, fortitude, and well-informed decision-making.

The book's provide a firm basis by extending a kind welcome and clarifying the aim of the work. The 'About the Author' section showcases the author's personal touch, which helps to build readership. This book provides a comprehensive overview of gallbladder cancer, including its definition, forms, occurrence, risk factors, symptoms, and the crucial role early discovery plays in the disease's treatment. This background information prepares readers to traverse the intricacies of diagnosis in this book, which covers diagnostic techniques, testing, and the cooperative role of medical experts.

The staging method is presented along with its implications for treatment options, prognosis, and survival rates. This is where understanding the stages of gallbladder cancer become critical. It explores several treatment modalities, including targeted therapies, immunotherapy, radiation therapy, chemotherapy, and integrative and complementary therapies. Giving people the skills they need to make educated decisions, stressing the importance of information, getting second opinions, and encouraging cooperation with medical teams are the main points of emphasis in Chapter 5.

The book offers assistance to individuals receiving treatment by discussing how to minimize side effects, provide emotional and psychological support, and stress the value of good nutrition and overall wellness. It also offers valuable perspectives on life beyond treatment, with a focus on follow-up care, survivorship, quality of life, and coping with recurrence.

Understanding the important role that caregiver's play, it is a special guide that looks at their roles, coping mechanisms, and helpful resources.

The book patient stories, which share real-life experiences and inspirational tales that offer hope, wisdom, and words of encouragement, give the story a poignant touch. The book ends with a discussion of advocacy and awareness, emphasizing the value of spreading knowledge about gallbladder cancer and promoting community involvement.

"Navigating Gallbladder Cancer with Confidence and Care" is essentially a lighthouse of support for those navigating the obstacles of gallbladder cancer. The book functions as a guide because of its well-structured layout and plenty of information; it provides not only a thorough grasp of the illness but also helpful suggestions, consolation, and opportunities for advocacy and awareness.

CHAPTER ONE

INTRODUCTION TO GALLBLADDER CANCER

KNOWING ABOUT COLORECTAL CANCER

The gallbladder is a tiny, pear-shaped organ that sits under the liver. Gallbladder cancer is an aggressive, comparatively uncommon type of cancer that starts there. Since symptoms of this kind of cancer may not appear until the disease has progressed to an advanced stage, early detection, and effective treatment are frequently extremely difficult. A thorough examination of this complex medical illness necessitates delving into several topics, including the description and forms of gallbladder cancer as well as its incidence, risk factors, symptoms, and the significance of early identification.

A SYNOPSIS OF BLADDER CANCER

An overview of gallbladder cancer starts with an appreciation of its basic characteristics. The storage and concentration of bile produced by the liver is a vital function of the gallbladder, an integral part of the digestive system. The gallbladder plays an essential role in the body, but it is also vulnerable to the growth of malignant cells that can cause gallbladder cancer.

The unchecked proliferation of aberrant cells in the gallbladder is the hallmark of this condition, which can have detrimental effects on general health.

DEFINITION AND TYPES OF CANCER IN THE GALLBLADDER

Examining the definition and various forms of gallbladder cancer reveals the intricacy of this illness. The most frequent type of gallbladder cancer is adenocarcinoma, although there are also less common variations such as squamous cell carcinoma and adenosquamous carcinoma.

Diagnosing and treating each subtype of cancer has distinct obstacles, highlighting the significance of having a comprehensive understanding of the cancer's particular characteristics.

RISK AND INCIDENCE FACTORS

Risk factors and incidence offer important new perspectives on the epidemiology of gallbladder cancer. Despite being a rare type of cancer, there are geographical variations in its prevalence, with some regions reporting higher rates than others. To determine who may be more likely to get gallbladder cancer, it is important to understand the risk factors linked to the condition. The entire risk profile is influenced by variables like age, gender, ethnicity, and specific medical disorders. This allows healthcare providers to apply focused screening and preventive techniques.

SIGNS AND TIMELY IDENTIFICATION

An essential part of treating gallbladder cancer is identifying its signs and stressing the value of early detection. Unfortunately, early on, symptoms are frequently evasive, delaying diagnosis and therapy start. Abdominal pain, jaundice, unexplained weight loss, and changes in bowel habits are common signs.

Healthcare professionals and the general public need to be more aware of these symptoms because early identification greatly enhances the prognosis and results of treatment for patients with gallbladder cancer.

A thorough comprehension of gallbladder cancer entails an intricate investigation of its description, classifications, prevalence, contributing components, and indications. Improving early identification and treatment options for gallbladder cancer is becoming more and more important as medical science and technology develop. Through a better understanding of this cancer, both medical professionals and the general public can help develop preventative, diagnostic, and management techniques that are more successful.

CHAPTER TWO

IDENTIFYING BLADDER CANCER

DIAGNOSTIC PROCEDURES AND TESTS

A thorough strategy involving a variety of diagnostic tests and procedures is required to diagnose gallbladder cancer. These are essential for detecting the existence of cancer, figuring out its stage, and creating a successful treatment strategy. A comprehensive medical history and physical examination are frequently the first steps in the diagnostic procedure, at which time medical staff members ask detailed questions regarding the patient's symptoms, risk factors, and general health.

A crucial part of the diagnosis process for gallbladder cancer is imaging testing. Often used to produce images of the gallbladder and its surroundings, ultrasound aids in the detection of any anomalies or masses. The precise cross-sectional pictures produced by computed tomography (CT) scans help determine the extent and spread of malignancy. To acquire fine-grained pictures of soft tissues, magnetic resonance imaging (MRI) can be utilized, providing important information about the properties of the tumor.

A biopsy is the most conclusive test for gallbladder cancer diagnosis. A tiny tissue sample must be taken out of the questionable area and sent for laboratory examination. This makes it possible for medical experts to identify the type of cancer, evaluate its grade of malignancy, and confirm its presence. Endoscopic retrograde cholangiopancreatography (ERCP) and percutaneous transhepatic cholangiography (PTC) are techniques that may be performed to collect biopsy samples and view the bile ducts.

THE VALUE OF TIMELY DIAGNOSIS

One cannot stress how crucial early detection is for gallbladder cancer. The chances of a successful intervention are increased and treatment results are markedly improved by early identification. A timely diagnostic workup is crucial since initial symptoms, such as jaundice and stomach pain, are nonspecific. Regular physical examinations and screening for people who have risk factors, such as a history of gallstones or persistent gallbladder inflammation, can help detect possible problems early on.

COLLABORATING WITH MEDICAL PROFESSIONALS

One essential part of the diagnosis process is collaborating with medical specialists. To guarantee a thorough assessment, a multidisciplinary team comprising radiologists, pathologists, gastroenterologists, and oncologists works together. While radiologists evaluate imaging information, gastroenterologists may perform endoscopic procedures. To choose the best course of action for treating gallbladder cancer, oncologists are essential in evaluating the disease's stage of diagnosis. By analyzing biopsy samples, pathologists offer vital information that helps the medical team comprehend the characteristics and activity of the malignancy.

Patients and medical staff must communicate with one another. Patients must communicate honestly with their healthcare staff about their symptoms, worries, and medical history. In addition to ensuring that the patient is educated about their ailment and the available treatment options, this collaborative approach promotes a more accurate diagnosis. Maintaining regular monitoring and follow-up sessions is also crucial to the management of gallbladder cancer since it enables medical personnel to evaluate the efficacy of treatment and swiftly address any new difficulties that may arise.

CHAPTER THREE

KNOWING THE GALLBLADDER CANCER STAGES

EXPLAINING THE STAGING SYSTEM

A staging system is frequently used to classify bladder cancer, assisting medical experts in determining the disease's extent and developing effective treatment strategies. The tumor's size, extent of invasion into neighboring tissues, and whether it has migrated to distant organs or lymph nodes are all commonly assessed as part of the staging system. The TNM (tumor, node, and metastasis) staging approach is widely applied to gallbladder cancer cases.

The "N" in the TNM staging system indicates if the cancer has spread to neighboring lymph nodes, the "M" indicates whether distant metastasis has taken place, and the "T" in the system reflects the size and extent of the initial tumor. The prognosis usually gets worse as the phases go from early to advance. Stages me through

IV show increasing tumor size and spread, while stage o denotes a very early, non-invasive malignancy.

EFFECTS ON AVAILABLE TREATMENTS

The selection of treatment options is largely influenced by the stage of gallbladder cancer. Surgery is frequently the main course of treatment in the early stages (I and II) of the disease when it is limited to the gallbladder and maybe surrounding tissues.

If the malignancy has spread to nearby organs, this may entail more involved operations or the removal of the gallbladder (cholecystectomy). To target any cancer cells that may still be present, further therapies like radiation therapy or chemotherapy may be suggested in some circumstances.

Treatment gets increasingly difficult as the cancer moves into stages III and IV. Advanced gallbladder cancer may invade distant organs, lymph nodes, or blood arteries.

Radiation therapy, chemotherapy, and surgery may be used in combination in certain instances. However, the main objective could change from treating the cancer to symptom relief, quality of life enhancement, and disease progression.

RATES OF SURVIVAL AND PROGNOSIS

Because gallbladder cancer is frequently diagnosed in its later stages, the prognosis is generally worse than that of certain other malignancies. The patient's general health, the stage of the cancer at diagnosis, and the effectiveness of treatment all have an impact on survival rates. Patients with an early diagnosis typically have a better prognosis than those with an advanced diagnosis.

The 5-year survival rate is comparatively greater for gallbladder cancer that is localized, or restricted to the gallbladder. However, survival rates usually decrease as the cancer spreads to distant organs or surrounding tissues. Stage IV gallbladder cancer typically has the worst prognosis because it has spread widely.

It is crucial to remember that survival rates are statistical averages and cannot be a reliable indicator of a person's fate. Patients with gallbladder cancer are experiencing increasingly better results thanks to developments in customized medicine and treatment options, and ongoing research is working to better understand the illness and develop future treatments that will be even more beneficial.

CHAPTER FOUR
METHODS OF THERAPY
OPTIONS FOR SURGERY

When it comes to treating a variety of illnesses, especially cancer, surgery is a basic therapeutic strategy. The goal of surgical procedures is to remove aberrant tissues or tumors from the body, either completely or partially. Many times, the location of the tumor, the patient's general condition, and the disease's stage all have a role in how well surgery goes. Options for surgery might vary from more involved open surgeries to less invasive techniques like laparoscopic procedures. Various procedures, such as organ removal, lymph node dissection, or tumor excision, may be used by surgeons depending on the patient's needs and the unique features of the disease.

CHEMOTHERAPY

Chemotherapy is a systemic treatment that targets and destroys rapidly dividing cells, such as cancer cells, using potent medications. This method works especially well for malignancies that have metastasized throughout the body. Chemotherapy medications can be infused intravenously or orally, and the treatment is frequently given in cycles to give healthy cells time to regenerate in between treatments. Even though side effects from chemotherapy can include nausea, exhaustion, and hair loss, research is still being done to create more focused and less toxic chemotherapy regimens that will improve treatment outcomes and patients' quality of life.

RADIATION THERAPY

To kill or harm cancer cells, strong doses of ionizing radiation are used in radiation therapy. Radioactive materials can be inserted directly into or close to the tumor to be administered internally, or they can be administered externally using devices that target particular bodily parts. Radiation therapy is often used in addition to or instead of surgery and chemotherapy as the main form of treatment. Because of its capacity to reduce tumor size, ease symptoms, and lower the risk of cancer recurrence, it is essential. Technological innovations like intensity-modulated radiation therapy (IMRT) and stereotactic radiosurgery keep improving radiation therapy's accuracy and efficacy.

IMMUNOTHERAPY

Immunotherapy is a novel form of treatment that stimulates the immune system to identify and eliminate cancerous cells. Drugs used in immunotherapy can improve the body's defenses against cancer by boosting the immune system. Among the many immunotherapeutic techniques are cytokine therapy, adoptive cell transfer, and checkpoint inhibitors. With some tumors, this method has demonstrated amazing efficacy, with some patients experiencing long-term remissions. Immunotherapy research is still in progress, to increase its effectiveness and broaden its range of applications to include more cancer types.

TARGETED THERAPIES

Targeted therapies aim to disrupt particular molecules that are essential for the proliferation and viability of cancer cells. Targeted therapies seek to specifically suppress cancer-related activities as opposed to standard chemotherapy, which affects both cancer and healthy cells. Small molecule medications or monoclonal antibodies that specifically target proteins or signaling pathways essential for tumor growth may be used in these treatments. By giving patients access to more potent and less toxic treatment choices, the discovery of targeted treatments has completely changed the way that cancer is treated. However, issues like medication resistance and the requirement for individualized treatment regimens continue to be the subject of ongoing research.

INTEGRATIVE AND COMPLEMENTARY THERAPIES

To improve their general well-being and control side effects from therapy, many cancer patients investigate integrative and complementary therapies in addition to traditional cancer treatments. These methods cover a wide range of treatments, such as mind-body techniques, dietary supplements, yoga, massage, and acupuncture. Even while these treatments might not directly attack the cancer, by attending to the patient's physical, mental, and spiritual needs, they can support the patient's holistic care. Complementary and integrative therapies are frequently utilized in addition to conventional medical treatments, and there is growing acknowledgment for their incorporation into all-inclusive cancer care programs. To learn more about the possible advantages and restrictions of these medicines in the context of cancer treatment, research is still being conducted.

CHAPTER FIVE

MAKING KNOWLEDGEABLE CHOICES

ACQUIRING KNOWLEDGE TO EMPOWER ONESELF

Knowing oneself is essential to make well-informed decisions, especially when it comes to healthcare. People have access to a multitude of tools in the information age that can help them comprehend their health conditions, available treatments, and possible consequences.

People can actively participate in health decision-making when they take the initiative to educate themselves about pertinent medical information. This empowerment promotes a feeling of control and makes it easier to have deeper conversations with medical providers.

People who are interested in learning more can look through credible sources including medical journals, trustworthy websites, and educational materials from healthcare organizations. A person is better able to have educated conversations with their healthcare providers when they are aware of the nuances of their disease, the many treatment options, and any possible negative effects. This cooperative method of decision-making establishes the groundwork for a more individualized and patient-focused healthcare encounter.

SEEKING REVIEWED WORKS

Getting second opinions is a wise and helpful strategy when making healthcare decisions. It recognizes the complexity of medical diagnosis and treatments, taking into account the fact that many healthcare providers may have different viewpoints. Getting a second opinion can provide people with a more comprehensive picture of their health condition and various perspectives on possible courses of treatment.

Getting second views is a proactive measure to make sure that decisions are thorough and well-rounded, not a reflection of mistrust toward a healthcare professional. They can be used to confirm a diagnosis, investigate different treatment approaches, or just get assurance on the suggested plan of action. People can make better decisions that fit with their interests, values, and general well-being by seeking out different points of view.

WORKING TOGETHER WITH YOUR MEDICAL TEAM

Working together with the healthcare team is essential to the decision-making process because it entails having candid conversations with a range of medical specialists. To provide comprehensive care, a healthcare team usually consists of physicians, nurses, specialists, and other support personnel, each of whom contributes their specialization.

Engaging in this cooperative endeavor enables people to express their aims, interests, and concerns, promoting a more customized approach to healthcare.

To collaborate effectively, one must actively listen to the opinions and suggestions of the healthcare team in addition to sharing one's views and preferences. With the help of this two-way communication, choices are made with a thorough grasp of the medical situation, accounting for the individual's specific needs as well as the clinical experience of the healthcare providers. By utilizing the combined knowledge of the healthcare team, collaborative decision-making supports a patient-centered care paradigm that upholds the autonomy and dignity of each individual.

CHAPTER SIX
MANAGING THERAPY
CONTROLLING ADVERSE REACTIONS

Overcoming the physical side effects of medical interventions is just one component of the complex process of coping with therapy. One very important part of this journey is managing side effects. Numerous medical procedures, like radiation or chemotherapy, can have a variety of adverse effects, ranging from exhaustion and nausea to changes in appetite and hair loss. Working collaboratively with healthcare providers to anticipate and manage these issues is a common component of coping methods. To minimize side effects and improve quality of life while undergoing therapy, people may benefit from alternative therapies, lifestyle changes, and medication.

MENTAL AND EMOTIONAL ASSISTANCE

Both psychological and emotional supports are crucial for negotiating the intricacies of medical care. When the physical requirements of treatment are added, the emotional toll of a diagnosis can be debilitating. A network of friends, family, and mental health specialists is often beneficial to patients.

There are spaces for people to share their hopes, worries, and anxieties through support groups and counseling programs. Prioritizing mental health in addition to physical health encourages resilience and aids people in navigating the emotional ups and downs that frequently accompany medical travel. Furthermore, mindfulness exercises like yoga and meditation may be very helpful in reducing stress and improving emotional health.

CONSUMPTION AND WELL-BEING DURING THERAPY

Well-being and nutrition throughout treatment are essential elements of a holistic care strategy. Keeping the body nourished becomes essential throughout therapy, as the body's nutritional requirements may change. Healthcare professionals and nutritionists frequently work together to create individualized meal plans that cater to the unique needs of each patient. Staying hydrated, eating a healthy diet, and taking supplements when needed will help keep the body strong and aid in its healing processes. Furthermore, when done according to medical professionals' guidelines, physical activity can enhance general wellness by boosting vitality and encouraging a sense of normalcy throughout treatment.

A comprehensive approach to coping is achieved by addressing the interrelated areas of emotional health, nutrition, and side effect management during therapy. By combining these ideas, it is acknowledged that mental and emotional healths are closely related to physical health. With the assistance of a cooperative healthcare team, patients are better equipped to handle the obstacles of their treatment, developing a sense of self-determination and fortitude in the face of hardship.

CHAPTER SEVEN
AFTER TREATMENT LIFE
AFTERCARE

Following the completion of cancer treatment, individuals often transition into a phase known as life after treatment, typified by a change from active medical treatments to a focus on recovering and preserving overall well-being. During this stage, follow-up care is essential. Scheduling routine follow-up consultations with medical professionals is imperative to oversee the patient's health and identify any possible indications of recurrence or long-term adverse effects. Physical examinations, imaging studies, and conversations regarding any lingering issues or symptoms may all be part of these appointments.

LIFE SPAN AND LIFE QUALITY

For those who have finished their cancer treatment, survival and quality of life become crucial factors. Being a survivor. involves more than just not having a sickness; it also involves an individual's overall health following treatment. It entails dealing with the social, emotional, and physical facets of life. Many survivors experience a mix of emotions, including relief, thankfulness, and occasionally dread due to the unpredictability of the future.

To help survivors transition and adjust to the obstacles of life after treatment, healthcare providers frequently play a crucial role.

Quality of life post-treatment comprises maximizing physical health and managing any lasting side effects or late-onset problems. The enhancement of the overall quality of life of cancer survivors may involve the implementation of rehabilitation programs, nutritional assistance, and psychological support. Not only is life expectancy stressed, but also the significance of leading a purposeful life after surviving cancer's obstacles.

HANDLING RECURRENCE

Even with the progress that has been achieved both before and after treatment, many survivors still have legitimate concerns about coping with recurrence. It can be emotionally taxing to fear that cancer will return, necessitating a careful balancing act between being vigilant and keeping a good mindset. A combination of continual medical monitoring, support groups and mental health services may be used as coping mechanisms. Promoting candid communication with medical professionals regarding any new symptoms or concerns is essential to swiftly addressing the likelihood of recurrence.

Every person's post-treatment path is different, depending on several variables including the kind and stage of their cancer, the therapy methods they received, and their level of personal resilience. The medical community is still working to improve survivorship care plans so that people entering this phase can receive comprehensive and customized support. Post-treatment can be a time of rekindled hope, fortitude, and the pursuit of a meaningful life beyond cancer with follow-up care, attention to survivorship, and successful recurrence management techniques.

CHAPTER EIGHT

A GUIDE FOR CAREGIVERS

THE CAREGIVER'S ROLE

When it comes to helping those who are unable to take care of themselves because of illness, disability, or aging, caregivers are crucial. Caregivers are responsible for a broad range of duties, such as assisting with everyday activities, giving medication, offering emotional support, and making sure the person they are caring for is healthy overall. Caregivers frequently act as vital liaisons between the healthcare system and the person receiving care, speaking out for their needs and arranging for different parts of their treatment to be coordinated.

In addition to providing physical care, caregivers also need to develop a sympathetic and reliable relationship with the person they are looking after. For the benefit of the care receiver as well as the caregiver, this emotional bond is essential. In addition, caregivers may have to schedule appointments, sort through complicated medical information, and help the care recipient and medical staff communicate. The dedication of caregivers is evidence of the significant influence they have on the lives of the people they look after.

HANDLING STRESS AS A CAREGIVER

Even though it can be satisfying, providing care can also be physically and emotionally taxing, which can cause stress or burnout in the caregiver. A caregiver's well-being may be negatively impacted by juggling a lot of obligations, seeing a loved one's health deteriorate, and coping with the uncertainties of caregiving. Caregivers must prioritize self-care and identify stress symptoms.

Setting reasonable goals for oneself and asking friends, family, or support groups for emotional help are two coping mechanisms for caregiver stress. Taking regular breaks, maintaining a healthy lifestyle, and utilizing respite care services can help a caregiver's overall well-being. Furthermore, seeking counseling or therapy choices and maintaining open lines of communication with medical professionals can be beneficial coping methods.

CAREGIVERS' RESOURCES

Various services and support networks are available to aid caregivers in their caregiving journey, acknowledging the difficulties they face. Caregivers can interact with others going through similar struggles by participating in online forums, support groups, and instructional workshops offered by local and national organizations. These platforms provide a forum for the exchange of knowledge, advice, and emotional support.

Practical resources including financial assistance programs, instructional materials on certain medical illnesses, and respite care services can be provided by government agencies, non-profit groups, and healthcare institutions. Caregivers ought to investigate these resources to broaden their understanding, obtain monetary assistance, and establish connections with experts who can offer counsel.

With the creation of apps and online tools to help with medication administration, appointment scheduling, and tracking health indicators, technology also plays a big part in aiding caregivers. By easing some of their logistical burdens, these services hope to free up caregivers to concentrate more on delivering high-quality care.

Caregivers play a variety of roles that include advocacy, emotional support, and physical caregiving. Maintaining a caregiver's well-being requires them to learn how to manage their stress, and there are many resources available to help them along the way.

CHAPTER NINE
AWARENESS AND ADVOCACY
THE SIGNIFICANCE OF LOBBYING

Promoting the rights and well-being of people and communities, solving societal concerns, and bringing about constructive change all depend heavily on advocacy. Its power to amplify voices, shape policy, and draw attention to urgent concerns that could otherwise go ignored accounts for its significance. Beyond awareness, advocacy is actively supporting and advancing a cause to effect real change. Through advocacy, people and organizations can promote diversity, influence policymakers, and build a society that is more just and equal.

INCREASING KNOWLEDGE ABOUT CANCER OF THE GALLBLADDER

One of the most important aspects of lobbying is spreading knowledge about certain health conditions; gallbladder cancer is one example. Despite being somewhat uncommon, gallbladder cancer can present significant health risks. In this case, the goal of advocacy is to raise awareness about gallbladder cancer's prevalence, risk factors, and symptoms. Through information dissemination, advocates work to promote early detection, diagnosis, and effective treatment for both the general public and healthcare professionals. Additionally, increasing awareness promotes communities that are supportive of persons affected by the condition and lessens the stigma associated with it.

PARTICIPATING IN THE COMMUNITY

Participating in the community is a great way to turn advocacy and awareness into concrete actions. Participation in the community creates a network of support that goes beyond individual endeavors by fostering a sense of shared responsibility and collective action. People can get involved in a variety of community-based projects, such as planning educational seminars on gallbladder cancer or holding fundraisers for organizations that support and further research. Through their active involvement in the community, advocates help to create a society that is more knowledgeable, caring, and resilient.

Involving the community means not just lending support to a cause but also establishing forums for discussion and cooperation. Advocates may foster a supportive environment that empowers those impacted by gallbladder cancer and their families by encouraging candid conversations and the sharing of personal experiences. The impact of advocacy and awareness campaigns is further reinforced by this sense of community, which fosters the sharing of information, tools, and emotional support.

The power of advocacy lies in its capacity to influence laws, create awareness, and encourage community involvement to effect positive change. When it comes to health problems like gallbladder cancer, advocacy is essential for enlightening the public, lowering stigma, and building support systems.